ACETAMINOPHEN: THE COMPREHENSIVE GUIDE

Understanding Acetaminophen, its Uses, and Safety Precautions

Dr. Acilino Morgan

Contents

CHAPTER ONE 4
- Introduction 4
- Origin of Acetaminophen 7
- Pharmacology of Acetaminophen: Understanding 15
- Uses of Acetaminophen 25
- Combination with Other Medications 31
- Dosage and Administration Guidelines 35
- Acetaminophen Overdose and Toxicity 38

CHAPTER TWO 39
- Causes of Overdose 39
- Symptoms of Overdose 42
- Overdose Treatment 44
- Long-Term Use and Chronic Effects 46
- Acetaminophen in Special Populations 51

CHAPTER THREE 58
- Dosage and Safety 58
- Alternatives to Acetaminophen 59
- Use in Older Adults 61
- Drug Interactions 65
- Acetaminophen and Public Health 66
- Regulation and Safety Measures 69
- Prescription Medications Containing Acetaminophen 70
- Reducing the Risk of Acetaminophen Toxicity 73
- Understanding the Mechanisms of Action 75
- Conclusion 81

THE END 85

CHAPTER ONE

Introduction

Acetaminophen, as it is known in the United States, or paracetamol as it is known in most of the rest of the world, is probably the most used medication in the world. It is taken to relieve pain and lower fever and thus is a mainstay of both the home medicine cabinet and institutional practice. Few individuals, however, have any knowledge of its history, mechanisms, therapeutic uses, and risks of its use. This book presents a critical review of acetaminophen, covering its discovery, pharmacology, its place in the practice of modern medicine, and the challenges brought about by its extensive application.

Origin of Acetaminophen

The history of acetaminophen began in the 19th century, at a time when scientists were vigorously involved in the hunt for a potent painkiller and antipyretic. During that era, treatment for painful conditions and fever was scant and attributed to poisonous remedies like opium, which had dangerous side effects. Researchers turned focus toward coal tar derivatives, the by-product of the industrial revolution, with hopes of finding possible medicinal uses for the substance.

In 1886, acetanilide was serendipitously discovered

when it had been given to a patient for intestinal worms, instead of naphthalene. Far from working on the worms, acetanilide lowered the fever of the patient, which set interest in the drug as a potential antipyretic and analgesic. It soon became apparent that acetanilide had serious toxic effects, among them methemoglobinemia, whereby hemoglobin is unable to release oxygen effectively to body tissues.

The researchers' next target was then phenacetin, a chemical very closely related to acetanilide but less toxic. Soon enough, phenacetin became the newest and most widely used pain reliever and fever reducer in the early 20th century. Much like its forerunner, however, phenacetin was also found to have appreciable adverse effects, particularly in causing renal damage and having a close link with some types of cancers.

The need for a safer alternative to phenacetin and acetanilide resulted in the discovery of acetaminophen, which was first synthesized in 1878 by American chemist Harmon Northrop Morse. Acetaminophen did not become prominent as an analgesic and antipyretic until the 1940s. It was shown that both acetanilide and phenacetin were metabolized in the body to acetaminophen, an active form of the compound responsible for therapeutic effects but lacking in the toxic side effects.

It was realized that acetaminophen was less toxic as compared to its predecessors, and by the middle of the 20th century, it had become so well known as an OTC drug. Its safe profile coupled with very efficient pain relief and antipyresis soon made it among the most popular drugs in the whole world.

Pharmacology of Acetaminophen: Understanding

Acetaminophen has been in wide use for years, but its mechanism of action has remained poorly understood. Unlike other nonsteroidal anti-inflammatory drugs like aspirin or ibuprofen, acetaminophen does not generally exhibit significant anti-inflammatory properties, hence complicating the explanation of its mechanism of pain relief.

The activity of acetaminophen is mediated primarily in the central nervous system. It has been shown to inhibit the enzyme COX (cyclooxygenase), which has a known role in the formation of prostaglandins—chemicals that cause inflammation, pain, and fever. However, acetaminophen has little effect on COX-1, which inactivates protective effects, such as stomach lining and kidney function processes, compared to other NSAIDs. This may explain the selectivity for why acetaminophen is less likely than other NSAIDs to cause stomach ulcers or kidney problems.

Recent studies have shown that acetaminophen can also enhance the activity in descending serotonergic pathways in the CNS, which modulate pain perception. Second, it can influence the endocannabinoid system to exert an analgesic effect.

Absorption: Acetaminophen is readily and quickly absorbed from the gastrointestinal tract following oral administration. Plasma peaks are usually seen within 30 to 60 minutes.

Metabolism: It is metabolized primarily in the liver through three main routes:

Glucuronidation: Acetaminophen undergoes conjugation with glucuronic acid to form an inactive metabolite.

Sulfation: Another fraction of acetaminophen is again conjugated with sulfate to form another inactive metabolite.

Oxidation: A small amount of acetaminophen gets oxidized by the cytochrome P450 enzyme system, mostly CYP2E1, to N-acetyl-p-benzoquinone imine, a highly electrophilic and possibly toxic compound.

Under normal conditions, NAPQI is inactivated by conjugation with the antioxidant glutathione to form a nontoxic compound excreted in the urine. In overdose, however, the amount of glutathione stored in the liver becomes too low to detoxify all of the NAPQI, which hence accumulates and causes hepatic injury.

In a healthy adult, acetaminophen has a relatively short half-life of 1 to 4 hours, which means it is flushed out from the body easily—hence, needs to be taken every 4-6 hours in order to be therapeutically active.

Due to its rapid absorption and metabolism, onset of action with acetaminophen occurs within 30 minutes to an hour, peaking for about 4-6 hours. This makes it quite suitable for acute symptoms of pain and lowering of fever.

Uses of Acetaminophen

Acetaminophen is one of the most used drugs for the relief of mild to moderate pain. Given its efficacy and safety, it is a first line of drug treatment for various painful conditions. These conditions include:

Acetaminophen is the drug of choice in tension headaches and mild migraines. It relieves pain without producing gastrointestinal side effects typical of NSAIDs; hence, it is preferable to many.

Acetaminophen relieves pain from muscle aches, joint pain, and back pain. This is very helpful for patients who cannot take NSAIDs due to gastrointestinal issues or other contraindications.

Acetaminophen is often prescribed for post-procedure pain control following dental procedures like extractions or root canals.

Acetaminophen combined with other analgesics is used to control post-surgical pain, especially in those situations where use of the NSAIDs is contraindicated.

Acetaminophen is mostly used in the alleviation of dysmenorrhea because of its analgesic effect and safety to be used for a prolonged period of time.

Acetaminophen is one of the most common antipyretics all over the world. It has shown great success in decreasing feverish conditions in both grownups and children, and usually, as recommended, it has a fine safety record.

Acetaminophen is an antipyretic of choice when it

comes to the treatment of fever in children, more so in those under six months. It is safer compared to aspirin, which is known to cause Reye's syndrome, a serious but rare condition in children. Acetaminophen is very commonly used in the management of vaccination-associated fever and discomfort in children and also in adults. Its efficacy in reducing fever without appreciable side effects has made it very popular in this application.

Combination with Other Medications

Acetaminophen is often combined with other drugs to enhance its actions or when the complaint involves multiple symptoms. The common combinations include:

Caffeine is added to acetaminophen in many over-the-counter preparations to prolong and enhance its analgesic actions, mainly for headache and migraine.

Acetaminophen is combined with an opioid—a drug such as codeine, hydrocodone, or oxycodone—in the treatment of more severe pain that might occur after surgery or from cancer. Treatment with these combinations should be taken with careful monitoring by a doctor because of increased risks of opioid addiction and acetaminophen toxicity.

Acetaminophen is another common component in multi-symptom cold and flu remedies. In such remedies, it is combined with decongestants, antihistamines, and cough suppressants. Such combinations may ease various symptoms like pain, fever, congestion, and coughing.

Dosage and Administration Guidelines

Acetaminophen is generally safe when used as directed. Usual adult dose: 500 to 1,000 mg every 4 to 6 hours; do not take more than 4,000 mg within a 24-hour period. However, to reduce the risk of liver damage, some experts recommend that the amount taken within a 24-hour period be limited to 3,000 mg, particularly in people at increased risk of liver damage.

Dosage is often calculated according to weight and age in children. This is why caregivers must use pediatric formulations of these products and follow the recommended dosing instructions on the label and as recommended by a doctor to avoid an accidental overdose.

Acetaminophen Overdose and Toxicity

One of the most harmful and dangerous acetaminophen-related risks is overdose, resulting in acute liver failure and sometimes even death. Acetaminophen overdose is the most common cause of acute liver failure in many countries, resulting from unintentional misuse.

CHAPTER TWO

Causes of Overdose

There may be overdose in several ways, including:

If taken well over the recommended dose, either

intentionally or unintentionally, the drug can overwhelm the liver's detoxification mechanisms for NAPQI, leading to hepatic toxicity.

Many over-the-counter drugs, as well as prescription drugs, contain acetaminophen. When people take more than one product containing acetaminophen unwittingly, an accidental overdose may occur.

Habits of taking more than the recommended amount over time can also build up toxic effects in the liver.

Symptoms of Overdose

Symptoms of an overdose of acetaminophen may not appear all at once, and they can include:

Nausea and Vomiting are the first signs of overdose. They can occur in a span of a few hours after taking the overdose.

Pain in the upper right quadrant of the abdomen is where the liver is located, this may likely point to damage to the liver.

With declining liver function, higher quantities of these poisons accumulate in blood and trigger confusion, drowsiness, and, finally, coma.

Yellowing of the skin and eyes is one of the indications that show very bad liver malfunction, meaning that one's liver is failing.

Overdose Treatment

If one overdoses on acetaminophen, he should be rushed to the hospital as quickly as possible. N-acetylcysteine works on the basis of increasing glutathione levels in the liver to rid it of NAPQI. For NAC to work optimally, it should be provided within 8 to 10 hours following overdose.

Those whose livers are severely damaged may be

forced to undergo a liver transplant to save their lives.

Long-Term Use and Chronic Effects

While acetaminophen is relatively safe in small quantities and during short-term use, concerns are emerging over some potential risks associated with long-term or high-dose use. Long-term intake of acetaminophen, especially near the maximum recommended daily dose, could bring about hepatic damage.

Another risk factor for acetaminophen-induced hepatotoxicity is chronic alcohol consumption, since ethanol induces the expression of the enzyme CYP2E1, thereby increasing the amount of the toxic metabolite NAPQI generated. People who have pre-existing liver conditions, such as hepatitis or cirrhosis, have an increased risk and should also be very careful while using acetaminophen under medical supervision.

Other studies also have suggested that, with long-term use at high doses, acetaminophen could be related to the damage of the kidneys, although this is considered less of a risk when compared to the NSAIDs.

Still, acetaminophen should be taken with caution by people with pre-existing kidney disease and under the supervision of their doctor.

Unlike NSAIDs, acetaminophen does not significantly affect the stomach lining or cause gastrointestinal bleeding.

However, chronic use, especially with high dosage intake, may still contribute to some risk towards the GI system, although the risk is very minor compared to those of NSAIDs.

Acetaminophen in Special Populations

Acetaminophen is thought to be one of the safest pain relievers and fever reducers for pregnant and breastfeeding women. However, as with any drug, it must be taken cautiously and only under the guidance of a healthcare professional.

Acetaminophen is considered safe at all stages of pregnancy. It forms the first line of treatment for pain and fever in pregnancy. This is because it does not involve exposure to gastrointestinal bleeding and other potential complications associated with NSAIDs. However, several studies have raised concerns regarding a potential association of acetaminophen use during pregnancy with an increased incidence of behavioural problems, like attention deficit hyperactivity disorder in children. Although these results are not conclusive, they indicate that acetaminophen should be used at the lowest effective dose and for the shortest duration possible during pregnancy.

Acetaminophen is known to be safe to take during breastfeeding. It passes into breast milk in very small amounts, which are not expected to cause harm to the infant. However, it is always prudent to consult with a healthcare professional before taking acetaminophen while breastfeeding.

Acetaminophen is a very common medication prescribed to children for pain and fever management. It is available in many formulations, such as liquids, chewable tablets, and suppositories, which make its administration relatively easy in children of varying ages and weights.

CHAPTER THREE

Dosage and Safety

Dosage is often based on weight and age in children. For this reason, using the correct pediatric formulation with proper dosing directions can help prevent accidental overdose. Overdosage in children can cause severe damage to the liver, so accurate measuring devices should be used, and the recommended dose should not be exceeded.

Alternatives to Acetaminophen

Acetaminophen is one of the widely used analgesics in

children to treat pain and fever. However, it can be substituted with other drugs such as ibuprofen if the child is old enough and in good health. Ibuprofen was claimed to possess anti-inflammatory properties absent in acetaminophen. Thus, it is highly effective in disorders or diseases where inflammation is implicated, such as in sprains or even in certain infections like ear infection. Nevertheless, ibuprofen must still be given to children with caution who are dehydrated or who have kidney problems.

Use in Older Adults

Acetaminophen is the most commonly used analgesic by older adults. It is particularly more widely used than NSAIDs in older patients, who are at increased risk for gastrointestinal bleeding, kidney damage, and cardiovascular events. Although acetaminophen is generally safer than these agents, there are some important considerations when it is used in older adults.

Liver function declines with increasing age, and this may impact the metabolism and clearance of acetaminophen. The elderly are at increased risk for hepatic toxicity resulting from acetaminophen, particularly if they have underlying hepatic disease or regularly consume alcohol. Older adults, however, can reduce this risk by only taking the lowest effective dose of acetaminophen and not exceeding the maximum recommended daily dose.

Drug Interactions

Older adults are likely to receive numerous medications that increase their risk of drug interactions. Although acetaminophen is reported to have lesser interactions compared to other analgesics, it remains vital to consult all medications with a healthcare professional to identify any potential interactions that can alter either the safety or efficiency of acetaminophen.

Acetaminophen and Public Health

Its wide availability as an over-the-counter drug makes it quite convenient for too many people to self-medicate for relief from pain and fever. However, the same wide accessibility also creates significant problems in terms of overdose and misuse risks related to public health. Enhancements to the labeling of acetaminophen-containing products have been forwarded to consumers, specifically regarding overdose risks and how not to exceed the recommended dose. There have also been educational campaigns to advise the general public on the risk associated with taking more than one acetaminophen-containing product at a time.

Regulation and Safety Measures

Some countries have restricted the quantity of acetaminophen that can be sold in a package, or have made the blister-packing of products containing acetaminophen, instead of selling them in bottles, to reduce the risk of inadvertent overdose. It tries to balance accessibility with protecting public health.

Prescription Medications Containing Acetaminophen

Besides being used as an over-the-counter drug, acetaminophen is often combined with an opioid in many prescription formulations for the relief of severe pain. While such formulations are often beneficial in controlling severe pain, they often lead to the addictions of opioids and frequently result in cases of acetaminophen toxicity.

The opioid crisis has cast an increased spotlight on the use of prescription pain medications that contain acetaminophen and opioids. There is increased awareness about the importance of good risk management in terms of such medications, including acute overdose of acetaminophen from patients who seek more pain relief than that indicated in the prescription.

Reducing the Risk of Acetaminophen Toxicity

Providers should strongly consider only prescribing the lowest effective dose of acetaminophen-containing medications and educate patients about the additional risks of taking acetaminophen from other sources. Some providers may wish to prescribe nonopioid alternatives or Spare the acetaminophen if more dosing flexibility is desired with the opioid component.

Understanding the Mechanisms of Action

Though acetaminophen has been in use for over a hundred years, not much has been clearly understood with respect to how it really works. Further research into the mechanisms of acetaminophen's analgesic and antipyretic actions may lead to a class of drugs with similar but more targeted benefits and fewer chances of adverse effects.

Safety and Efficacy: Enhancement

Research is also targeted on increasing the safety and efficacy of acetaminophen.

This involves investigating new formulations that could reduce the risk of overdose and examining potential antidotes or protective agents that could be used in cases of overdose.

Acetaminophen and Chronic Pain

Recent interest is growing in understanding the role that acetaminophen can play in the management of chronic pain. While acetaminophen is often used to treat acute pain, its efficacy and safety for chronic pain are less well understood.

The study in this area may help further elucidate its role in the long-term management of pain and help to identify possible associated risks of chronic use.

As public health agencies continue to grapple with the challenges presented by acetaminophen overdose and misuse, there is a need to continually research effective prevention and education strategies. This ranges from the study of the impact of regulatory changes and public awareness campaigns, among other interventions that might reduce instances of acetaminophen-related harm.

Conclusion

Acetaminophen has been one of the mainstays of medicine in recent history, partly due to its effectiveness in analgesia and antipyresis but also because of its relatively modest side effect profile when used appropriately. Its broad and sometimes indiscriminate use, along with easy over-the-counter availability, presents significant issues with overdose and hepatic toxicity.

THE END

THE END

www.ingramcontent.com/pod-product-compliance
Lightning Source LLC
Chambersburg PA
CBHW070205230526
45471CB00002B/834